Anti - Inflammatory Diet Cookbook For Begginer

50+ Recipes To Help Reduce Weight And Fight Against Chronic inflammation

Ivy Dennis

Copyright - Notice

All right reserved. This book or any portion thereof may not reproduce or used in any manner whatsoever without the express written permission of the publisher.

No part of this book maybe reproduced, or stored in a retrieval system, or transmitted in any form or by any means, electronic,mechanicals,recording,or otherwise, without express written permission of the owner.

Table of contents

Chapter - One

Introduction

The mainstay of an anti-inflammatory diet Cookbook is fresh produce, which is rich in antioxidants. Foods contain compounds known as dietary antioxidants that aid in the body's elimination of free radicals. Naturally occurring byproducts of several body functions, such as metabolism, are free radicals.

Inflammation manifests as discomfort, redness,swelling,heat, and loss of function. The body's intricate biochemical reaction to damaging stimuli, including irritants, infections, and damaged cells, includes inflammation.

 You may experience no symptoms at all or feel hot or lose function due to inflammation in your body's cells or tissues. Inflammation may lead to additional tissue damage and illness if it doesn't go away on its own and becomes persistent.

Reduced blood pressure, improved mental and cognitive performance, and relief from various chronic conditions can all be achieved with an anti-inflammatory diet. Additionally, since processed foods and refined sugars are frequently higher in calories, you'll consume fewer of them.

Chapter -Two

Component Parts Of A Healing Plate

The Primary Elements

Nutrients are necessary for all living things to thrive and to grow and develop appropriately. The elements (components) of food known as nutrients give us the nutrition we need to survive. In addition to giving our bodies energy, nutrients support the growth and maintenance of organs, tissues, bones, and teeth. They also help control bodily processes including blood pressure and metabolism. Vitamins, minerals, protein, carbs, and lipids are examples of nutrients.

 The patient's nutritional needs and limits will be specified in the Care Plan, which will give guidance to an HHA/PCA. As these are set up to best support the patient's health, Home Health Aides and Personal Care Aides should always make sure to abide by them. If they are ever uncertain as to whether a patient is eligible to consume a certain food, they should consult their supervisor for advice.

We are overloaded with food alternatives every day, which makes it challenging to select the healthiest options. Because processed meals are more widely available, individuals have faster lifestyles, and their diets often consist of convenience foods deficient in important nutrients. Therefore, it is impossible to overestimate the significance of whole foods in our daily nutrition. We'll explore what whole foods are, why including them in your diet is beneficial, and helpful advice for starting the transition to healthier eating habits in this extensive book.

An increase in processed foods

Whole foods were the main diet of most people in the past. Yet more processed foods are being produced as a result of advances in food science technology. A lot of sugar, salt, trans fats, and non-nutritive, artificial substances are frequently found in these items, all of which are harmful to human health.

How Does a Whole Foods Diet Work?

Foods that have been minimally processed or altered are referred to as whole foods. They have returned as closely as feasible to their former state. Plant foods like as fruits and vegetables, whole grains, legumes, nuts, and seeds are among them; some animal foods like fish, poultry, and dairy products are also included.

Qualities of complete foods Among entire foods' primary characteristics are:

Rich in nutrients: Rich in fiber, vitamins, minerals, and health-promoting phytonutrients

Not overly sophisticated: little altered from their original composition or combined with unreal substances.

little amount of additives Low or no added salts, sugars, artificial colorings, or preservatives.

 Whole food examples

Whole foods include, for instance:

Fruits and vegetables: Broccoli, carrots, apples, oranges, berries, and so forth

Whole grains include quinoa, brown rice, oatmeal, and whole wheat bread.

Legumes: kidney beans, black beans, chickpeas, and lentils, among others.

Nuts and seeds: Flaxseeds, chia seeds, sunflower seeds, walnuts, almonds, etc.

Lean proteins include fish, tofu, eggs, turkey, chicken breast, and so forth.

Dairy: cheese, milk, yogurt, etc.

The significance of fresh produce

Essential vitamins, minerals, and plant compounds can be found in fruits and vegetables. They have fiber as well. Fruits and vegetables come in a wide range of kinds, and there are numerous methods for preparing, cooking, and serving them. Consuming a lot of fruits and vegetables can help ward off heart disease, diabetes, and cancer.

Chapter - Three

<u>Strong protein</u>

A diet rich in protein is necessary for good health. Beyond its vital functions in constructing and preserving human tissues and muscle, as well as in assisting with the regulation of numerous bodily functions, protein also aids in the promotion of satiety, or fullness, and may help with weight management.

Thankfully, there are plenty of lean protein sources, both plant and animal-based, to help you reach your target.

What foods are low calorie but high in protein?

Foods that are high in protein but don't have a lot of calories or fat include legumes, low-fat dairy, as well as lean meats, fish, or plant proteins like tofu, or quinoa, which has around 8 grams of protein and only 2.5 g of fatTrusted Source in 1 cooked cup.

What is the best protein with the lowest calories?

Fish and beans have the least amount of calories per 100 g while also containing 8-28 g of protein depending on the food.

How do I get 150 g of protein a day?

A balanced, nutritious diet will include enough protein to fulfill the 150 g recommendation. Lean animal proteins include white-fleshed fish, skinless poultry, and cuts of red meat such as loin and round. Low fat dairy products, like cottage cheese, yogurt, and milk are also good sources of protein. Plant proteins like beans, tofu, and powdered peanut butter offer ample protein too.

Which foods are high in protein but low in calories?

Foods that are high in protein yet low in calories or fat include fish, legumes, low-fat dairy products, lean meats, and plant proteins like tofu or quinoa, which has about 8 grams of protein and only 2.5 grams of fat.In one cooked cup, a reliable source.

Which protein has the most calories and the finest quality?

With 8–28 g of protein per 100 g, depending on the item, fish and beans offer the fewest calories per 100 g.

How do I obtain 150 grams of protein each day?

Protein should make up no less than 150 grams of a well-balanced and nutrient-dense diet. White-fleshed fish, skinless chicken, and cuts are examples of lean meats.

Chapter - four

Healthful fats

Omega-3 Fatty Acids: A Crucial Amount

The majority of the fats required by the human body can be produced by the body from other fats or carbs. For omega-3 polyunsaturated fatty acids, often known as omega-3 fats and n-3 fats, that isn't the case. These fats are necessary; the body cannot produce them on its own; food is the only source. Nuts (particularly walnuts), flax seeds, leafy vegetables, various vegetable oils, and some types of fish and seafood are foods high in omega-3.

Why are omega-3 fats unique? They influence how the cell receptors in these membranes function and are necessary for the construction of cell membranes throughout the body. They also serve as the precursor for the synthesis of hormones that control inflammation, artery wall contraction and relaxation, and blood clotting.

Omega-3 types

The two primary forms of omega-3 fats that are vital to human health are as follows:

DHA and EPA: Also known as marine omega-3s, docosahexaenoic acid (DHA) and eicosapentaenoic acid (EPA) are primarily found in cold-water fish. High-quality sources of EPA/DHA include sardines, mackerel, tuna, herring, and salmon. It would be more accurate to refer to EPA and DHA as "conditionally essential" fats as they can be produced from alpha-linoleic acid (ALA), another omega-3 fat. However, it is recommended to get EPA/DHA straight from food sources because the conversion from ALA to these fats may not be effective enough.

ALA: The most prevalent omega-3 fatty acid in most Western diets, alpha-linolenic acid (ALA) can be found in nuts (walnuts, chia, and flax seeds), plant oils (canola, soybean, and flax), and nuts.

Four Healthy Fats to Eat Each Week

Avocado: Avocado is a superfood that is packed with healthy monounsaturated fats. In addition to being a great source of healthy fats, avocados are also loaded with vitamins, minerals, and fiber. Adding avocado to your diet is an easy way to improve your overall health.

Nuts: Nuts such as almonds, walnuts, and cashews are a great source of healthy fats. They are also high in protein, fiber, and antioxidants. Nuts are a convenient snack that can be enjoyed on their own or added to meals such as salads or oatmeal.

Fatty fish: Fatty fish such as salmon, mackerel, and sardines are an excellent source of omega-3 fatty acids. Consuming fatty fish on a regular basis can help reduce inflammation, improve brain function, and reduce the risk of heart disease.

Olive oil: Olive oil is a healthy source of monounsaturated fats. It is also rich in antioxidants and anti-inflammatory compounds. Using olive oil as your primary cooking oil is an easy way to add healthy fats to your diet.

In conclusion, healthy fats are an essential component of a balanced diet. Consuming healthy fats can help reduce your risk of heart disease, lower blood pressure, and improve brain function. Incorporating healthy fats into your diet is easy and delicious. Try adding avocado, nuts, fatty fish, and olive oil to your meals each week to reap the benefits of these healthy fats.

Four Good Fats to Consume Every Week

Avocado: Rich in beneficial monounsaturated fats, avocados are a superfood. Avocados are a fantastic supply of good fats and are also a terrific source of vitamins, minerals, and fiber. Including avocados in your diet is a simple approach to enhance your general well-being.

Nuts: Almonds, walnuts, and cashews are a few types of nuts that are a fantastic source of good fats. They also include a lot of fiber, protein, and antioxidants. Nuts are a handy snack that go well with salads or oatmeal, or they can be eaten on their own.

Fatty fish: A great source of omega-3 fatty acids is fatty fish, like sardines, mackerel, and salmon. Regularly consuming fatty seafood can help lower it.

Chapter - Five

Bright recipes full of antioxidants

Antioxidants are substances that may aid in delaying or even preventing the body's cellular deterioration. Plant-based meals include a wide range of antioxidants, including beans, cocoa, green leafy vegetables, blueberries, and cocoa. Antioxidants may aid in protecting the body from potentially dangerous free radicals that can cause oxidative stress.

Which four antioxidants are examples of?

Examples of antioxidants include vitamins C and E, selenium, and carotenoids including lutein, zeaxanthin, lycopene, and beta-carotene.

The Top 12 Antioxidant-Rich Foods

Apples.

Berries and avocado.

Chocolate.

veggies that are cruciferous.

Verdant Tea.

Specifically, mushrooms.

nuts.

What fruit contains the most antioxidants?

blueberries

Antioxidants are found in large amounts in a variety of plant foodsq, but they are concentrated in red and purple fruits such as raspberries, blackberries, pomegranates, tart cherries, blueberries, and goji berries.

Super Berry: It keeps you from aging too soon because to its amazing concentration of antioxidants.

With its combination of dietary fiber, phytosterols (lipid-like molecules derived from plants), and monounsaturated (healthy) fats, açaí is a powerful tool for supporting digestive and cardiovascular wellness.

What health benefits might berries provide?

Berries are a good source of potassium, magnesium, fiber, vitamins C and K, and prebiotics, which are carbohydrates that support a healthy gut flora.

Antioxidant dietary recommendations

veggies as well as beans or legumes, fruit,

wholegrain cereals and meals. lean beef, chicken, or tofu, fish, eggs, lentils, nuts, and seeds as substitutes.

dairy and dairy substitutes, primarily low-fat varieties (milk with lower fat content shouldn't be given to babies younger than two years old).

Smoothie bowls are simply thickened smoothies with added nutrients that can be eaten with a spoon. They are frequently garnished with nuts, seeds, fruits, muesli, or oats. McKel Hill, MS, RD, is the author of the plant-based, whole foods blog Nutrition

Stripped. "Think of smoothie bowls as the new cereal -- like cereal 2.0."

Because smoothie bowls are heavy in natural sugars and fiber, they improve satiety, aid in better digestion, and maximize the absorption of all nutrients. It also prevents infections, improves bowel movements, strengthens immunity, maintains a healthy heart, and generally improves quality of life.

While "eat the rainbow" offers some excellent nutritional advice, "taste the rainbow" is a reference to Skittles advertisements. (Of course, assuming the rainbow you're eating isn't composed of Skittles.)

The various hues of fruits and vegetables are linked to specific vitamins and antioxidants. This implies that you will be consuming a wide variety of nutrients if your meal contains every color of the rainbow. In addition to being really delicious, a rainbow smoothie bowl is the ideal way to get extra nutrition into your breakfast.

Did we also mention that it's simple? With just a few minutes of preparation the night before, you can have this smoothie bowl ready in the morning!

ABOUT THIS SMOOTHIE BOWL, RAINBOW

Spoon it out and eat it. Smoothie bowls have an easy concept. You will make your smoothie somewhat thicker so that it can be consumed with a spoon rather than making it a drinkable smoothie. You can also top your smoothie with a lot of toppings and not worry about them sinking to the bottom of the bowl thanks to this thicker volume!

Simple to alter. Consider this rainbow smoothie bowl to be somewhat similar to a breakfast ice cream sundae. Make sure to employ a rainbow of colors while customizing your smoothie foundation by adding whatever toppings you desire!

Chapter - Six

Meals that cure the stomach

What do probiotics entail? When applied or taken by the body, probiotics—live microorganisms—are supposed to provide health advantages. They're present in beauty products, dietary supplements, and

fermented meals like yogurt and others.

Here are some naturally occurring probiotic-containing fermented foods and ideas for serving them to your family.

Kefir and yogurt made from milk or nondairy milks like soy, coconut, and water...

Pickles, kimchi, and sauerkraut.

Miso, tamari (soy), tempeh (soy), kombucha, and so on.

aged cheese, cottage cheese, and sour cream

At what point are probiotics advised?

Your healthcare practitioner may suggest probiotics if you experience dysbiosis symptoms, whether they be in your digestive system or elsewhere, in order to help restore balance to your microbiome. In the event that you lately became ill or If your microbiome was compromised by a treatment, your doctor may provide probiotics to help restore it. For instance, they might advise utilizing or taking probiotics following the completion of an antibiotic course.

A daily probiotic supplement is something that some people use to keep themselves healthy overall. If you find that it helps and you are prone to gut health difficulties, you might want to try this. In addition to lowering inflammation and supporting regular bowel movements, a healthy gut flora can strengthen your immunity overall. Probiotics are one way to Aid in the restoration of your gut flora, which can be diminished by daily factors like stress and eating choices.

Which probiotics work well?

In order for a probiotic to be beneficial to your health, it needs to choose a verity that has been shown to boost your health.

Exist in a form that is safe for your body to apply or ingest.

Risks / Benefits

What are the potential health benefits of probiotics?

The beneficial microbes that live in different parts of our bodies assist us in a variety of ways. One of the most important ways is by fighting off the more harmful types of bacteria 8, fungi, viruses and parasites that might also want to live with us. Probiotics, in theory, fight on the side of your beneficial microbes.

Many probiotic products are formulated with beneficial bacteria and yeasts for the purpose of preventing or recovering from bacterial or yeast infections in your different body parts, including:

Benefits / Risks

What possible advantages do probiotics provide for your health?

The helpful microorganisms that inhabit various body areas provide us with several benefits. Keeping out the most dangerous strains of bacteria, fungi, viruses, and parasites that could wish to coexist with humans is one of the most crucial strategies. Theoretically, probiotics defend your good microorganisms in the struggle.

Beneficial bacteria and yeasts are added to many probiotic products in order to help prevent or treat bacterial or yeast infections in various body areas, such as:

.acne as well as atopic dermatitis.

. gum disease as well as cavities.

. urinary tract infections (UTIs) and vaginal infections.

. diarrhea linked to antibiotics

 Recipes for the following :

Yogurt - Six Essential Steps for Making Yogurt at Home

The milk should be heated to 180 degrees Fahrenheit.

Lower the milk's temperature to between 112 and 111.5 °F.

Add the beneficial bacteria that is your yogurt starter.

Mix the remaining milk with the yogurt beginning.

Transfer the milk into jars and let it sit for seven to nine hours.

To cool and solidify, put the jars in the refrigerator.

Kimchi - Start by preparing two heads of napa cabbage for this recipe. Adding taste, extending the shelf life, and removing excess moisture from the cabbage are all achieved by rubbing it with coarse sea salt. Fish sauce, garlic, white sugar, ground ginger, green onions, and white onions are also required.

Start by preparing two heads of napa cabbage for this recipe. Adding taste, extending the shelf life, and removing excess moisture from the cabbage are all achieved by rubbing it with coarse sea salt. Fish sauce, garlic, white sugar, ground ginger, green onions, and white onions are also required.

Kombucha - A fermented beverage created with tea, sugar, yeast, and bacteria is called kombucha tea. First, a culture of yeast and bacteria must develop in order to produce the beverage. The tea and sugar are combined with the culture.

Chapter - Seven

Spices and herbs with taste

Certain spices and herbs, such as black pepper and ginger, have anti-inflammatory properties that can improve your general health by reducing inflammation.

The body uses inflammation to combat infections and promote recovery.

But occasionally, inflammation can get out of control and persist longer than is necessary. This is known as chronic inflammation, and research has connected it to a number of illnesses, such as cancer and diabetes.

Your diet is very important to your health. Your diet, especially different types of herbs and spices, can impact inflammation in your body.

The science underlying nine spices and herbs that may reduce inflammation is reviewed in this article.

It is noteworthy that inflammatory indicators are molecules that are discussed in numerous studies in this text. These suggest that inflammation is present.

Therefore, a plant that lowers blood levels of inflammatory markers also probably lowers inflammation.

Garlic

The well-known spice garlic (Allium sativum) has a potent flavor and aroma. For thousands of years, people have utilized it in traditional medicine to treat a variety of conditions, including toothaches, infections, constipation, arthritis, and coughs (6Trusted Source).

Garlic's sulfur-containing components, including S-allylcysteine, diallyl disulfide, and allicin, are mostly responsible for its health benefits and seem to have anti-inflammatory qualities (7Trusted Source, 8Trusted Source, 9Trusted Source).

A comprehensive review of 17 high-quality trials spanning 4–48 weeks and involving over 830 participants revealed that supplementing with garlic significantly lowered blood levels of the inflammatory marker CRP (10Trusted Source).

Nonetheless, aged garlic extract shown greater efficacy in lowering blood levels of TNF-α and CRP (10Trusted Source).

Ginger Zingiber officinale, or ginger, is a flavorful spice that is both sweet and spicy. There are several methods to use this spice: powdered, dried, or fresh.

In addition to its culinary applications, ginger has been used for thousands of years in traditional medicine to treat a wide range of illnesses. Colds, headaches, nausea, arthritis, and elevated blood pressure are a few of them (1Reliable Source).

More than 100 active chemicals, including zingiberene, zingerone, shogaol, and gingerol, are found in ginger. These are probably in charge of its health benefits, which include assisting the body in reducing inflammation (2Trusted Source).

Taking 1,000–3,000 mg of ginger daily for 4–12 weeks significantly reduced markers of inflammation when compared with a placebo, according to an analysis of 16 research involving 1,010 people.

Ground Turmeric

Turmeric, or Curcuma longa, is a spice that has been used for ages in Indian cooking.

It contains more than 300 active ingredients. The main one is curcumin, an antioxidant with strong anti-inflammatory properties (13Trusted Source).

Numerous studies have shown that curcumin can suppress the activation of NF-κB, a protein that activates genes that cause inflammation (14Trusted Source, 15Trusted Source, 16Trusted Source).

1,223 people who took 112–4,000 mg of curcumin daily for three days to thirty-six weeks were studied in a review of fifteen outstanding trials (17Reliable Source).

The administration of curcumin significantly reduced inflammatory markers when compared with a placebo. Interleukin 6 (IL-6), high-sensitivity C-reactive protein (hs-CRP), and malondialdehyde (MDA) were some of the markers (17Trusted Source).

Southeast Asians are the original producers of cardamom (Elettaria cardamomum). It tastes complex, peppery, and sweet.

According to research, ingesting supplements containing cardamom may help lower inflammatory markers like MDA, TNF-α, IL-6, and CRP. Moreover, a study discovered that cardamom increased antioxidant status by 90% (23, 24, 25, 26, 26 Trusted Sources).

In an 8-week trial involving 80 prediabetic participants, it was discovered that ingesting 3 grams of cardamom daily, as opposed to a placebo, dramatically decreased inflammatory markers such hs-CRP, IL-6, and MDA (23Trusted Source).

Similarly, 3 grams of cardamom or a placebo was given daily to 87 individuals with nonalcoholic fatty liver disease (NAFLD) for a duration of 12 weeks (24Trusted Source).

The levels of the inflammatory markers hs-CRP, TNF-α, and were much lower in those who took cardamom.

A tasty and aromatic plant native to the Mediterranean region is rosemary (Rosmarinus officinalis).

Studies indicate that rosemary may be useful in lowering inflammation. This is thought to be because of the high concentration of polyphenols it contains, including carnosic acid and rosmarinic acid (43Trusted Source, 44Trusted Source).

Compared to a placebo, a 16-week research involving 62 individuals with osteoarthritis found that consuming a daily tea high in rosmarinic acid significantly decreased pain and stiffness and enhanced knee mobility (45Trusted Source).

Rosmarinic acid was found to decrease inflammation indicators in both animal and test-tube trials related to a variety of inflammatory disorders, including as gum disease, asthma, osteoarthritis, and atopic dermatitis (46Trusted Source, 47Trusted Source, 48Trusted Source, 49Trusted Source).

Vinegar and oils infused with herbs are excellent ways to enhance the flavor of your food. They are simple to prepare and go well with salads, marinades, and pasta sauces, among other foods. The best part is that you may alter them to your preference and try out various herb and flavor combinations.

The sort of herbs you use while creating herb-infused oils and vinegar can have a significant impact on the finished product's flavor and aroma. Here are some of the greatest herbs to use in your own herb-infused oils and vinegar, along with some recipe ideas to get you started and usage advice.

A wonderful present, infused oil is somewhat of a gourmet delight. Excellent quality olive oil is the key to creating delectable infused oils. Top-notch olive oil: Read our best suggestions for selecting the perfect product if you need assistance. Your recipient will like the gorgeous and delectable infused olive oil that Wildly Organics' olive oil fulfills all of the requirements for.

This is the recipe for cold-infused rosemary oil that you may make. As soon as you master the art of infusing olive oil with rosemary, you may experiment with different herbs and spices, such as thyme or basil, or even chiles or garlic powder. Upon mastering the fundamental methods, you can create an assortment of infused oils. Alright, let's go!

How to go about It

Making rosemary oil in a slow cooker is fantastic, but if you don't have one, the cooktop method works just as well.

Cooktop Rosemary Extract

Assemble the components.

The Spruce Eats gathered the ingredients for the recipe for rosemary oil.

Use a pot that is hefty and warms up evenly. Avert aluminum and cast iron that isn't enameled. Pour the oil over the rosemary that has been placed in the pot.

Leaves of rosemary in a pot

The Spruce Consumes

Heat for five to ten minutes on low heat. The oil should warm up but not simmer.

Place oil and rosemary in a pot over the fire.

The Spruce Consumes

After turning off the heat, leave the oil with the rosemary infusion for one hour.

In a saucepan over low heat, add the oil and rosemary.

What The Spruce Consumes

Fill a clean, dry glass container or jar with the strainer (this recipe doesn't require the bottle or jar to be sterilized). Tightly cover and refrigerate for a maximum of 10 days.

Rosemary oil in a storage jar with a swivel top.

Chapter - Eight

little amounts of carbs

Grains are the seeds of grasses grown for food. These plants also are called cereals. Examples of grains include wheat, oats and rice. Each grain, also called a kernel, is made of three parts:

Bran. Bran is the hard outer coating of a kernel. It has most of the kernel's fiber. It also has vitamins and minerals.

Germ. The germ is the part that sprouts into a new plant. It has many vitamins, healthy fats and other natural plant nutrients.

Endosperm. The endosperm is the energy supply for the seed. It mostly contains starches. It has small amounts of proteins and vitamins. The endosperm has very little fiber.

What nutrients are in whole grains?

The bran from any kind of whole grain is a good source of fiber. Nutrients in whole grains vary. They may include the following nutrients and others:

Vitamin A.

Vitamin B-1, also called thiamin.

Vitamin B-2, also called riboflavin.

Vitamin B-3, also called niacin.

Vitamin B-6, also called pyridoxine.

Vitamin B-9, also called folate.

Vitamin E.

Iron.

Magnesium.

Phosphorus.

Selenium.

Grains are the edible seeds of grasses. Cereals is another name for these plants. Grains include things like rice, wheat, and oats. A grain, often known as a kernel, consists of three components:

Bran. The tough outer layer of a kernel is called bran. It has most of the fiber from the kernel. Minerals and vitamins are also present.

Pathogen. The portion that develops into a new plant is called a germ. It's packed with vitamins, good fats, and other organic plant nutrients.

endosperm. The seed receives its energy from the endosperm. Starches make up the majority of it. Vitamins and proteins are present in trace levels. There is hardly any fiber in the endosperm.

How to increase the amount of whole grains you eat

For additional whole grain in your meals and snacks, try these suggestions:

Savor whole-grain cereals for breakfast, such as oatmeal, shredded wheat, or whole-wheat bran flakes.

Instead of ordinary bagels, try whole-wheat toast or whole-grain bagels. Instead of pastries, try whole-grain, low-fat muffins.

Utilize whole-grain rolls or breads to make sandwiches.

Instead of using white-flour tortillas, use whole-wheat tortillas.

Make use of wholegrain pastas.

Use brown rice, wild rice, bulgur, barley, or other grains in place of white rice.

In salads, casseroles, stews, and soups, use barley or wild rice.

To give ground beef or poultry more body, mix in healthful grains such cooked brown rice or whole-grain breadcrumbs.

In place of dried oats, use crushed whole-wheat bran cereal or rolled oats.

You'll obtain more nutrients that are good for your health if you eat a range of whole grains. Adding variety to your meals and snacks also helps them become more fascinating.

 Notes on nutrition: quinoa, brown rice, and sweet potato recipe -

This recipe yields a healthy dish! It might be difficult to obtain whole grains that are devoid of wheat or gluten for those who must avoid wheat because of a wheat allergy or intolerance.

Quinoa is a special kind of whole grain, more like a seed. It delivers a complete protein in addition to fiber and B vitamins. It therefore includes all nine of the necessary amino acids, which are not produced by our bodies.

Compared to most grain dishes, this one has a higher protein content—roughly 6 grams per serving.

A portion of this dish will also provide you with a good amount of fiber! In addition to being whole grains and excellent providers of fiber, quinoa and brown rice also include some fiber from the veggies.

DIRECTIONS:

Set oven temperature to 350°F. Apply cooking spray to an 8-quart casserole dish.

In a big skillet, warm the oil over medium heat. Saute the sweet potato, onion, carrot, and celery in the skillet until they are soft.

Add the quinoa, brown rice, stock, thyme, and salt to the 8-quart casserole dish after scooping in the sautéed veggies. Mix everything together.

Bake for 30 to 40 minutes, or until the grains are soft and the liquid has been absorbed, in a preheated oven. Serve right away.

Chapter- Nine

<u>Medicinal teas</u>

Turmeric, ginger, chamomile, and peppermint teas are a few teas that can aid with inflammation reduction. Because these teas have anti-inflammatory qualities, they may aid in lowering bodily swelling.

Given that tea has been utilized for millennia as a natural treatment, its discovery that it possesses anti-inflammatory qualities comes as no surprise. Although inflammation is the body's normal reaction to damage or infection, persistent inflammation can cause a number of different health issues. Tea use can help lower inflammation and enhance general health.

There are a few considerations to make while selecting the finest tea for inflammation. To start, seek out teas that have anti-inflammatory ingredients like flavonoids and polyphenols. Second, think about your favorite kind of tea. Herbal teas, black teas, and green teas each offer special tastes and health advantages. The tea's origin and quality should be your last consideration.

Olinda Turmeric, Ginger, and Ginseng Herbal Tea is a fantastic option if you're searching for a flavorful tea that also reduces inflammation.

The combination of turmeric and ginger is perfect for reducing inflammation and increasing energy levels.

Olinda teas are made with high-quality ingredients and are heavily influenced by Ayurvedic culture, making them a great choice for overall wellness.

Olinda is a carbon-neutral and sustainable tea company, so you can feel good about your purchase.

Cons

Some may find the taste of turmeric and ginger to be too strong.

The tea bags are not individually wrapped, which may be inconvenient for some.

The price point is slightly higher than other similar teas on the market.

We were pleasantly surprised by the taste of this tea, which was both flavorful and soothing. The combination of turmeric and ginger is perfect for reducing inflammation, and the addition of ginseng helps to increase energy levels. We also appreciated that Olinda teas are made with high-quality ingredients and are heavily influenced by Ayurvedic culture, making them a great choice for overall wellness.

Advantages:

Turmeric and ginger work wonders together to boost vitality and decrease inflammation.

Olinda teas are an excellent option for general wellbeing because they are created with premium ingredients and have a strong Ayurvedic influence.

Olinda is a sustainable and carbon-neutral tea brand, so you can buy with confidence.

Ayurvedic Loose Leaf Tea with a delicious flavor that supports digestion and the immune system is SOLA Organic Anti Inflammatory Ayurvedic Loose Leaf Tea.

Advantages:

Turmeric, ginger, lemongrass, and licorice root combine to provide a potent anti-inflammatory mixture.

The tea has no added sugar or preservatives and is brewed with premium organic ingredients.

The format of loose leaf tea enables a brewing experience that is adjustable.

Cons

For people who are not accustomed to the taste of ginger or turmeric, the tea may be quite strong.

It could take a little longer to prepare loose leaf tea than tea bags.

Certain tea infusers or cups may become stained due to the tea's yellow hue.

Ginger-Turmeric Lemonade

This lemonade is cold, crisp, delicate, and spicy all at once. It doubles as a great hot tea as well; simply reheat it and savor!

Ingredients

four and a half cups water

1 1/2-inch piece of raw ginger, diced, peeled.

1 1/2-inch piece of raw turmeric, cut, peeled, and

two tsp honey

one and a half tablespoons lemon juice

A pinch of black pepper

UNIQUE EQUIPMENT

Blender

Fine-mesh bag or nut-milk strainer

Peeler for vegetables

DIRECTIONS

In a high-speed blender, combine water, ginger, turmeric, lemon juice, honey, and black pepper; mix until smooth.

Blend the ingredients with a sieve.

Just like you would with homemade broth, skim the foam off the top.

Serve immediately over ice or chill.

NOTES ON THE RECIPE: Upon sitting motionless, a thin sediment will settle at the bottom of the drink container. For quick shaking before serving, a mason jar makes the perfect storage container.

Chapter - Ten

Useful advice for regular cooking

What does cooking meal planning entail? is the process of planning meals ahead of time based on your preferences, timetable, available foods, seasonal produce, sale goods, etc. As a result, weekly grocery shopping for only the necessities is usually the result of meal planning, with the help of others (like family) to help create the menu. Meal planning and batch cooking are undoubtedly related, although they employ slightly distinct techniques. Meal planning can be as simple as knowing what's for dinner every night or as complex as organizing a week's worth of meals and cooking them all at once.

Conversely, batch cooking involves preparing the ingredients for several meals at once. It's possible that you'll use the ingredients you produced during batch cooking in the meals you've scheduled for yourself each week, Batch cooking also play a big part in the planning of a meal.

Steps to Plan Your Meals

Determine your goal. First things first, you want to determine your goal. ...

Calculate your daily energy needs. Next you'll need to calculate your daily energy needs. ...

Divide daily energy (calorie) needs into meals and snacks. ...

Write down your meals for the week or next few days. ...

Go food shopping.

How to Take Into Account the Elements in Meal Planning

Meeting Nutritional Needs.

Addressing Allergy and Lifestyle Concerns.

Maintaining Your Budget.

Verifying the Ingredient and Resource Availability.

How to Schedule Your Meals

Establish your objective. foremost things foremost, you need to decide what your objective is.

Make a daily energy needs calculation. The next step is to figure out how much energy you'll require each day.

Organize your daily energy requirements (calories) into meals and snacks.

Put your meals for the upcoming week or several days in writing.

Visit a grocery store.

Food that is organic or purchased from a pricey health food store is not necessary to reduce inflammation. Actually, some of these have undoubtedly been in your kitchen for a long time.

Most chronic diseases, including diabetes, cancer, and heart disease, are caused by chronic inflammation; however, inflammation can often be treated without the use of medications. You can use food to combat inflammation.

The good news is that you don't have to eat organic, pricey, or uncommon foods to combat inflammation. You are also not required to visit specific establishments or sign up for monthly deliveries. In fact, you most likely already have a few staple anti-inflammatory foods in your freezer, fridge, or pantry.

See this list of the top 7 kitchen essentials that reduce inflammation.

1. Herbs

While it may seem that pungent spices and dried herbs could worsen inflammation, evidence reveals that they have the opposite effect. In reality, other cultures have long utilized its aromatic components for therapeutic purposes due to their anti-inflammatory properties. Although turmeric is frequently mentioned, other dry herbs and spices that also have anti-inflammatory properties include ginger, cinnamon, cumin, and rosemary.

2. Based on legumes Pasta

Since they first hit the shelves about ten years ago, pastas made with flour from lentils, fava beans, and chickpeas have become increasingly popular. These legume-based pastas are higher in protein, fiber, and other nutrients when compared to refined and whole-grain varieties. This promotes fullness and blood glucose control, but it also facilitates the preparation of a high-protein, meatless spaghetti supper. Additionally, eating a few vegetarian meals each week reduces inflammation.

3. Tomatoes in Cans

While they are a fantastic source of potassium, vitamin C, and folate, it's the phytochemical lycopene that makes tomatoes stand out among other anti-inflammatory foods. Tomato products that are boiled or have had minimum processing are excellent sources of lycopene, which lowers inflammation linked to heart disease and cancer. In actuality, lycopene content in tomato pastes, sauces, juices, and other canned goods can be up to five times more per cup than in fresh tomatoes.

4. Berries that are frozen

Fresh produce frequently lacks anti-inflammatory ingredients compared to that which is flash-frozen soon after harvest. This is because once collected, fruits like strawberries and blueberries have the highest concentration of nutrients; but, after that, they gradually lose their vitamins and minerals.

However, freezing can stop that loss. For a powerful dose of antioxidants and anthocyanins that can help to reduce inflammation both now and in the future, frozen berries are therefore perfect to have on hand in the freezer.

5. Salmon or tuna in a can

Most of us don't consume nearly enough omega-3 fatty acids on a weekly basis, despite research suggesting that they provide some of the best anti-inflammatory benefits. But having a few cans or pouches of tuna, salmon, or other fish in the pantry is one of the simplest ways to start making this happen. These kinds of cold-water fish are among the few healthy food sources of omega-3s, so make an effort to eat them two or three times a week.

6. Tea Drinking a cup of black or green tea every day may help to decrease the beginning and progression of Alzheimer's disease, increase the growth of beneficial bacteria in the stomach, and reduce or block the production of cancer cells. Studies indicate that these benefits are due to catechins, which are anti-inflammatory chemicals found in tea. If you also drink

other caffeinated beverages, choose green over black and monitor your total intake.

7. Eggs

Eggs are a fast, high-quality source of protein that are always in the refrigerator but are simple to forget. Additionally, they are among the top providers of choline and selenium, two nutrients that reduce inflammation.

Actually, half of each person's daily demands are met by two eggs. Additionally, some people discover that eating a lower-carb breakfast—such as eggs—helps them control their blood sugar levels throughout the day. This is significant because frequent blood sugar rises and falls are linked to elevated inflammation.

Conclusion

Enjoy good health

Reaching your fitness or other health-related goals can be facilitated by starting small, concentrating on one behavior at a time, and getting encouragement from people.

Once more, you're driven to adopt the healthier lifestyle you've been promising yourself, including improving your diet, increasing your activity, cutting back on your caffeine intake, and more. You've tried previously and most likely made a New Year's resolve to try again, but you didn't feel very successful.

It can be difficult to change your lifestyle, particularly if you want to do a lot of changes at once. This time, consider it a progression rather than a conclusion.

Making changes to one's lifestyle is a process that needs patience and assistance. The hardest part of making a change is deciding to stick with it once you're ready. Thus, plan ahead and conduct thorough study to ensure your achievement. Planning carefully entails establishing minor objectives and moving slowly.

For long-lasting, constructive lifestyle and behavior changes, consider the following three suggestions:

1. Create a strategy that will work. Your plan serves as a road map to help you navigate this journey of change. It's even

possible to consider it an adventure. Be detailed in your plan creation. Do you want to work out more? Describe the best time of day to go for walks and the distance you plan to go. Put everything on paper and ask yourself if you are sure that these pursuits and objectives are within your reach. If not, begin with more modest measures. As a reminder, post your strategy where you'll see it the most.

2. Modify one conduct at a time. It takes time to replace harmful behaviors with good ones since unhealthy behaviors build up over time. When people try to change too much too quickly, they

frequently encounter difficulties. Aim for one goal or change at a time to increase your chances of success. Try incorporating a new objective that contributes to the overall transformation you're aiming for as soon as your new, healthy behaviors become second nature.

3. Include a friend. Someone else on your journey, be it a friend, colleague, or relative, will help to keep you accountable and inspired. Maybe it will be someone who joins you at the gym or someone who is also attempting to give up smoking. Discuss the work you are doing. Have a look at joining a support

group. Working on the mission becomes less daunting and the work itself easier when you have someone to share your achievements and problems with.

Starting a health journey involves a lot of hard work, dedication, and perseverance. It's critical to pause and acknowledge your accomplishments as you move closer to your objectives. Celebrating your accomplishments not only lifts your spirits but also serves to reinforce the good behaviors you've formed along the road. This post will discuss five fulfilling ways to recognize and celebrate your health journey accomplishments, which will keep you encouraged and motivated to keep moving forward.

1. Put together a physical challenge
Putting together a fitness challenge is one of the most fun ways to commemorate your accomplishment in your health journey. Organize a fun competition with your friends, family, or even coworkers. It could be a collective exercise, a race, or a team sport. This will serve as a reminder of your journey's accomplishments as well as a means of fostering healthy rivalry and companionship.

2. Invest in a Spa Day for Yourself
A pampering spa day is the ideal approach to treat yourself after a successful endeavor. Make an appointment for a massage, facial, or any other rejuvenating treatment that will help you relax. In addition to reducing your physical tension, the pampering experience will allow you to celebrate your achievements and recognize the importance of self-care in your overall health journey.

3. Arrange an Exciting Adventure

Arrange an adventurous and vigorous celebration of your health achievements. Hiking a beautiful trail, riding a bike through a new city, or trying out an exhilarating outdoor sport like rock climbing or kayaking are a few examples. Taking part in these experiences not only offers a distinctive and thrilling experience, but it also serves as a reminder of the power and talents you have acquired along the way.

4. Take Pictures to Document Your Development

One way to remember your health journey would be to schedule a professional photo session. Wear things that accentuate your growth and give you a sense of confidence. Whether you take pictures by yourself or with your loved ones, having a physical record of these occasions will show you how far you have come. Others who might be beginning their own health journeys may find inspiration in the images.

5. Acquire a New Ability

Celebrate your path toward better health by broadening your horizons and picking up a new skill. Enroll in a fitness session, talke up dancing classes, or sign up for a cooking class that interests you. Learning a new talent will not only be

fulfilling, but it will also increase your
self-esteem and keep your attention
focused on your general well-being.

I